I0118643

Our Others Keeper (OOK) is built from an idea of servitude and giving. I firmly believe that we must do all we can to take care of one another.

My mother....

My brother...

My neighbor...

I am *Our Other's Keeper*

Thank you

Thank you for purchasing a My Portion nutritional program cycle. I am excited to begin this journey with you.

I am grateful for you.

Authentic success is being so grateful for the many blessings bestowed on you and yours that you share your portion with others.

~Sarah Ban Brethnach

What is "My Portion" program

~ The **My Portion** program is foundational to addressing health and wellness goals. My Portion is designed to appreciate your uniqueness and use that to help you easily reach your goals. No one does everything wrong and you have been alive this long without dying... ☺ What this program is designed to do is to help you make informed decisions about the food you consume on a daily basis that will help you reach nutritional goals.

The nutritional goals support the physical goals...in case you are not sure where I am going with this.

~ Think about the idea that "Abs are made in the kitchen." Does your diet support you having abs....maybe not yet but it is possible REGARDLESS of who you are. Everyone has something they really like to eat: Some are healthy and some are not so healthy. But we can work together one cycle at time to direct your thinking towards the healthier options. Yes, there are different steps that need to be taken to achieve "abs" if that is your goal but we can work through these steps together.

My Portion is STEP # 1.

Where are you now?

~ Before we begin with Step # 1, the nitty gritty of the program, it is important that you define where you are and where you want to go. I am here to support you! You got this!

~ On the following page, I would like you to attach a picture of yourself...one that you really like. This picture should be a picture that most accurately represents you in everyday life. This is a snapshot of what you look like and how you feel. If you don't love the way you look in your picture, address the areas that you would like to change to make it "perfect".

Headshots are not going to work. This is a nutritional wellness program after all....

~ Before you attach your picture write how you are feeling in your current body. Write in **exactly** what you would like to improve and a reason for wanting that improvement.

~ Next, get that tape measure and fill in the blanks.

Start..........

Before:
I feel......
I want to improve.....
Because....

This is me on _____(date).

I recommend that you attach a printed picture

Arms

Mid section

Lower body

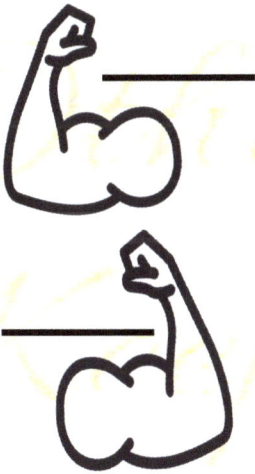

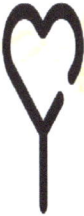

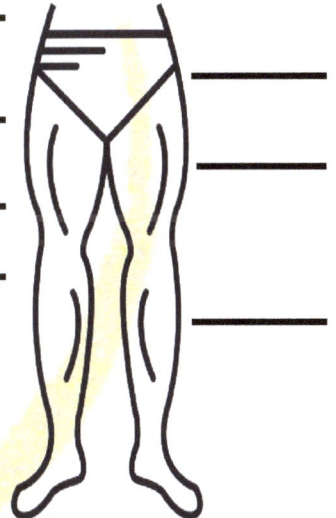

"Icon made by FreePik from www.flaticon.com"   "Icon made by FreePik from www.flaticon.com"   "Icon made by FreePik from www.flaticon.com"

MORE
DATA

Ok by now, you are either extremely excited about getting started because this is seeming too easy to be true or you're a little disheartened by how you are looking and feeling. Either way....

You are amazing and you will make significant changes to your health and wellness.

I believe in you.

~ Two websites that are used to provide me information on how to help you build your My Portion cycle is:

Precision Nutrition Calculator Once you get to the brief summary screen record that information on the following page. You can click the available link to get a **free complete guide** and this is the information that I need and will use to build your cycle starting point.

Grocery store online cart/list I personally use Kroger.com. I decide on the items that will last me approximately 2-3 weeks and I put these in a list or cart. One reason that I love doing this online is because I can see the amount of money that I am spending.

Sometimes my budget does not allow me to eat 2 pounds of Salmon and high quality grass fed beef.

~ Complete this task and send me the list/cart. Remember you **only** eat what you put in this cart and we are going to decide on changes based on your specific needs. Think this through!

For Your Information...

Here are some tips for building your list/cart of food.

1 ~ Write out recipes that you are good at making and love to eat

2 ~ Find recipes online that you would like to try based on your diet preference. (Keto, Paleo, Vegan, etc..)

3 ~ List snacks and drinks that you routinely consume.

This is the hardest part of this plan. Feel free to reach out to me if you need additional support in this area.

Precision nutrition calculator
Brief Summary

~ Feel free to print a screenshot of your brief
summary and attach it here instead of
writing the information in. ~

Current weight _____

Eating Style _____

Macro Percentages

_____Calorie

_____Protein

_____Carb

_____Fat

GOALS

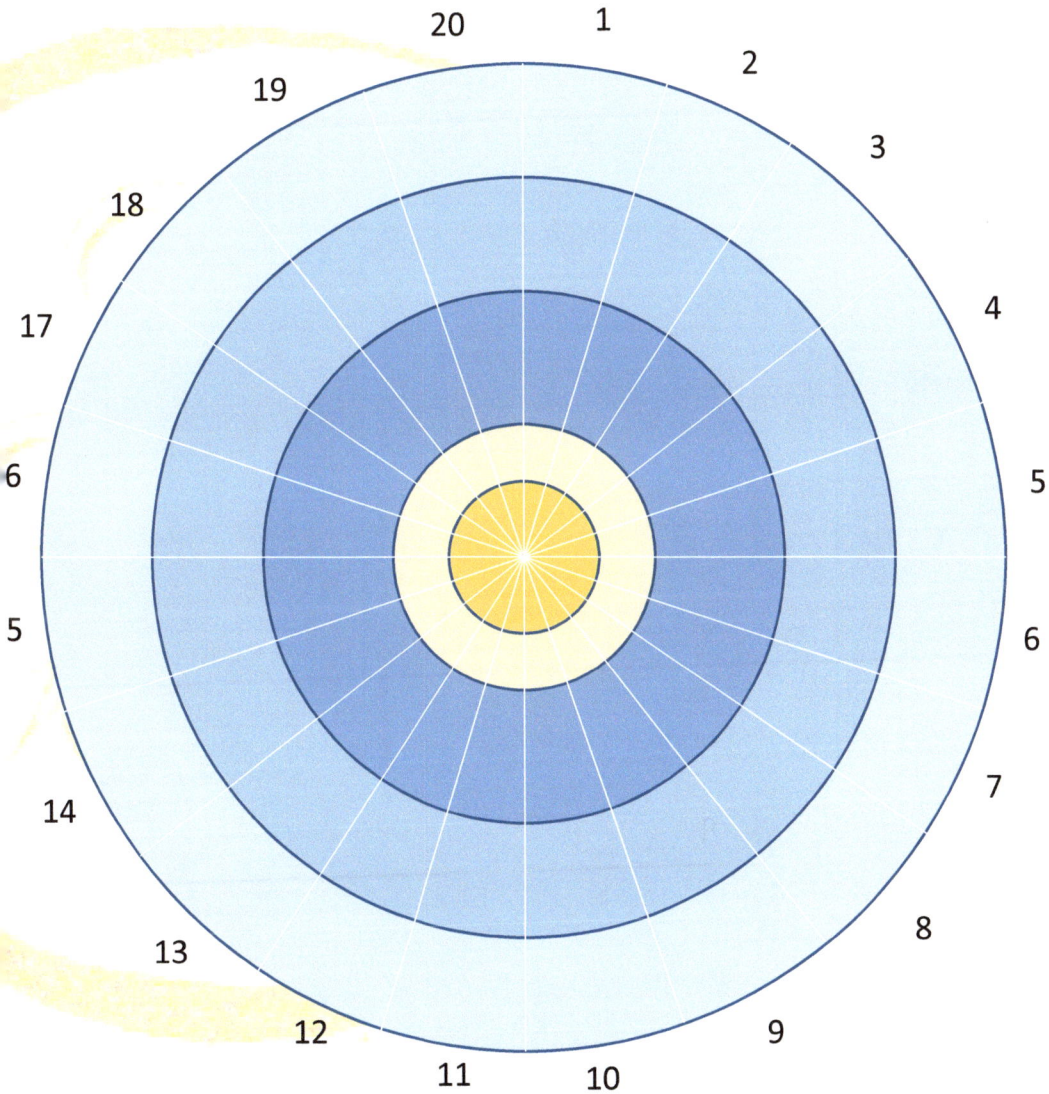

Goals Legend

On the goals page, Color in your goals day by day as you meet them.
*Write in your goals below**

☐	_____
☐	_____
☐	_____
☐	_____
☐	_____

For this cycle of nutrition training, what are your goals.

~Remember that we should not exceed 2 pounds per week, if weight loss/gain is your goal~

~ For this plan, I asked that you made a grocery list of items that you usually consume in a 2-3 week period. Majority of grocery stores in my area offer delivery and pickup services after purchasing items online. Personally, I am all for this because I looooove going to the grocery store. The sales, the smells, the samples.... I usually want everything and spend way more money than I intended to because of the amazing marketing that I experience in the store.

~ The best way to curb the temptation of poor choices is to begin online. You are more than welcome to use the list you create to go into the store to purchase the items after we adjust for your needs.

A friend of mine absolutely refuses to buy fruits and vegetables without first putting them through her rigorous quality standards: Squeezing and sniffing.

~ What are your nutritional goals?

~ What are your physical / body goals?

~ Are there any upcoming events in the next 2-3 weeks that may prevent your success on this plan?

Maybe you are thinking, if I eat the same things I have been eating, won't my weight just stay the same?

My Portion plan is designed around what you eat and what you like.

~ When I initially began my STRONG journey on January 1, 2020, I followed the usual training model of being given or assigned meals that supported muscle gain but I HATED it! Let me tell you why. There are foods that I like and eat often and there are foods that I don't like or don't eat very often. Rice is an example of the latter. I very rarely eat rice. On plans that I have allowed others to develop for me, there was almost always an inclusion of ½ cup of rice, quinoa, or some other carbohydrate....

<u>The problem with this is most grocery stores do not sell rice by the ½ cup.</u>

What am I going to do with a bag/box of rice that I have only used a ½ cup from? The answer is ...... Eat it.

If a food is in your house or possession, either you, someone you love, or someone you marginally tolerate, will eventually eat it.

~Berardi's First Law

Strategy
or
Tragedy

I **do not** like wasting food and I definitely **do not** like wasting money.

When choosing foods for the 2-3 week time span, you have to give this a little thought.

Can you handle yourself in the kitchen?

What can you make?

Have you seen a recipe lately that you would like to try?

Are there 3-5 dishes that you are really good at making that can be considered your "go-to" staples?

~ For me, I absolutely love to cook and to meal-prep. My friends think I am OCD about it but....well, maybe I am.

~ There are several wonderful dishes that I love to consistently make. I love smoothies, morning breakfast wraps, and Enchiladas. I tailor my plan to things that I will eat because I like them.

There is a lot less temptation to stop at a drive-thru when I know I have enchiladas at home.

This section is called Strategy or Tragedy because I went through it.

I developed this plan.

I believe in this plan.

I have learned so much about myself from this plan.

~ As I mentioned before, I love enchiladas and would make them every cycle if my nutrient guide allowed it. The very first time I made the Keto Enchiladas, I planned out 3 portions for an 11 day cycle. The first fork full ended that plan. I devoured **ALL** of them. The kicker is I wasn't even that hungry. I just *really really* liked the way that they tasted.

For the remainder of the cycle, I was SAD!

~ After that my lesson was learned. Even though, this plan allows you all of the freedom you need to be successful, you must remember to listen to and OBEY your fullness cues, reign in going overboard when you are dealing with challenges outside of your plan, and plan out your portion so that you always have access to success. Freedom to choose can be your strategy or your tragedy.

My Portion program is a transformation system designed around the way that you prefer to eat. You make the diet plan, you consistently follow the diet plan, you reach your goals!!!

Keep going with...

An upcoming grocery list
Precision Nutrition Macro calculations
A completion mindset
and......
Patience

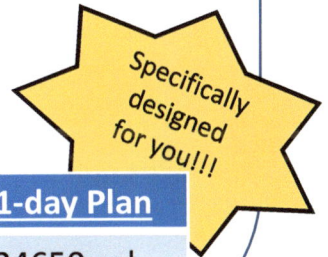

Specifically designed for you!!!

Macro Targets	Daily	21-day Plan
Calories	1650 cal	34650 cal
Fat (g)	138 g	2888 g
Carbohydrate (g)	33 g	693 g
Protein (g)	56 g	1178 g

Macro breakdown example for a 21 day plan.

21 day plan Outline - Example

~ The following page is an example of a 21-day plan I created for myself using ingredients that I routinely purchase at my local grocery store. Everything on my plan is something that I love to eat and can use in several different recipes. I shop based on recipes that I like and have meal-prepped a dozen or more times before. I purchased glass dishes with lids, smoothie glass bottles, coffee cups, and a few other things that make meal prep super easy and convenient for me.

Remember! This is your plan so you need to make arrangements to take steps for you to be successful. If you need more in-depth work on analyzing trends and patterns following this first cycle, please feel free to schedule a consultation with me for additional cycles addressing your long-term goals.

~ In this plan outline, you can see the food items that I ate. Working out is optional until your nutritional foundation is built and can be incorporated as you advance in future cycles.

BIG FACTS

Your plan may look
nothing like my plan.

Your exercise regimen
may look nothing like
my regimen.

This plan is designed for
you and only you.

21 Day Plan Example

Day # 1	Day # 2	Day # 3	Day # 4	Day # 5	Day # 6	Day # 7
Food	**Food**	**Food**	**Food**	**Food**	**Food**	**Food**
Eggs Creamed spinach Meatballs Smoothie	Sweet and Savory faux griddle Smoothie	Eggs and Bacon Broccoli soup with cauliflower rice Smoothie	Eggs Salmon cucumber sandwiches Smoothie	Spinach wrap with ham and cheese Smoothie	FASTING	Eggs and avocado Smoothie Enchiladas Chicken and Spinach
Exercise	**Exercise**	**Exercise**	**Exercise**	**Exercise**	**Exercise**	**Exercise**
Upper	Mid-Lower	Upper	Active Recovery or rest	Mid-Lower	Active Recovery or rest	STRONG by Zumba
Weight ___	**Weight** ___	**Weight** ___	**Weight** ___	**Weight** ___	**Weight** ___	**Weight** ___
Day # 8	Day # 9	Day # 10	Day # 11	Day # 12	Day # 13	Day # 14
Food	**Food**	**Food**	**Food**	**Food**	**Food**	**Food**
Breakfast wrap Veggies stuffed cheese wrap Meatloaf and sweet potato Smoothie	Salmon and green beans Breakfast wrap Smoothie Rebel Ice Cream	Beef stuffed peppers Breakfast wrap Veggies stuffed cheese wrap Smoothie	Enchiladas Breakfast wrap Avocado egg salad in lettuce Smoothie	Salmon and green beans Eggs and Kielbasa omelets with cheese Rebel Ice Cream	Beef Stuffed peppers Breakfast wrap Veggie stuffed cheese wrap Smoothie	Ravioli Breakfast wrap Smoothie Keto ground beef casserole
Exercise	**Exercise**	**Exercise**	**Exercise**	**Exercise**	**Exercise**	**Exercise**
Upper	Mid-Lower	Upper	Active Recovery or rest	Mid-Lower	Active Recovery or rest	STRONG by Zumba
Weight ___	**Weight** ___	**Weight** ___	**Weight** ___	**Weight** ___	**Weight** ___	**Weight** ___
Day # 15	Day # 16	Day # 17	Day # 18	Day # 19	Day # 20	Day # 21
Food	**Food**	**Food**	**Food**	**Food**	**Food**	**Food**
Eggs and avocado Smoothie Meatloaf and sweet potato	Breakfast wrap Cabbage and Kielbasa Smoothie	Ravioli Breakfast wrap Smoothie Keto ground beef casserole Rebel Ice Cream	FASTING	Thai noodle soup Veggie stuffed cheese wrap Eggs and Avocado	Veggie stuffed cheese wrap Cabbage and Kielbasa	Thai noodle soup Veggie stuffed cheese wrap
Exercise	**Exercise**	**Exercise**	**Exercise**	**Exercise**	**Exercise**	**Exercise**
Upper	Mid-Lower	Upper	Active Recovery or rest	Mid-Lower	Active Recovery or rest	STRONG by Zumba
Weight ___	**Weight** ___	**Weight** ___	**Weight** ___	**Weight** ___	**Weight** ___	**Weight** ___

TIME TO BUILD YOUR PLAN

~ Now that you have completed the Precision Nutrition Calculator and created a grocery list of things that you like:

1 ~ Submit that information to me

2 ~ Schedule coach time to discuss how to make positive changes

3 ~ Agree to follow the plan and not deviate

4 ~ Grocery shop for the items you have selected.

Weigh and account for all of the food.

This is to double check the macro calculations and solidify the reasonable time frame for this portion cycle of food. Sometimes I cannot always get what I planned and have to make changes.

Usually, the plans are **10-21** days.

This allows for food to be consumed without going bad and prevents boredom.

To support you in the My Portion program, you will receive:

❑ A cycle plan outline with the number of days, calories, and macros in a calendar format.

❑ A documentation journal to track your progress. *Journal includes an intermittent fasting table (advanced clients), water accountability, a "to do" section, a workout focus, and a workout log.*

❑ Weekly check-ins with me to address issues that may arise. If you begin the plan on a Monday your check-in day is Sunday.

From this point, there is no calorie counting, no weighing food, no restrictions other than eating what is on the plan and nothing more.

I suggest that you print 2 copies of your My Portion plan. One copy is to post in your kitchen and the other copy is to keep with you throughout the day. Both of these copies are to serve as a reminder to not deviate from the plan. You have decided on your success and now all you need to do is be successful.

Not done yet

~There are things that I purchased that are not in the nutrition calendar. These things are used for those times when I need a little more food that what I planned.

~This plan is to focus on what you consider a portion size. If you experienced any "tragedies" like I did with the enchiladas then you now have better insight on your eating habits.

~This plan should last you for the entire duration of the cycle. If you ran out of food – that is a portion control issue. If you have food left over – you are not eating enough.

JOURNAL

Day # 1 _____

Nutrition Plan

Window	Item	Calories	Fat (g)	Carb (g)	Fiber (g)	Protein (g)
Fasting 4am – 11 am	Green tea with Lemon					
Feeding 11am – 7pm	Eggs Creamed Spinach with meatballs Smoothie					
Fasting 7pm – 4am	Green tea with Lemon					
Fasting _____						
Feeding _____						
Fasting _____						

EXAMPLE

Last Bite Eaten @

Water

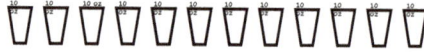

120 oz.

TO DO LIST

_____

_____

Workout Focus

Chest	Arms	Back	Glutes	Shoulder	Abs	Rest
✓	✓	✓		✓		

Workouts in Reference

I am so grateful for movement

Workout Log

Exercise	Minutes	Reps	Weight	Sets
Elliptical	25	1		3
Barbell bench press		4-6		3
One Arm dumbbell row		4-6		3
Standing military press		4-6		3
Barbell Curl		4-6		3
Tricep Kickback		4-6		3

Note

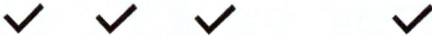

_____

_____

_____

_____

_____

_____

_____

_____

Day # 2 _____

Nutrition

Window	Item	Calories	Fat (g)	Carb (g)	Fiber (g)	Protein (g)
Fasting 4am – 11 am	Green tea with Lemon					
Feeding 11am – 7pm	Eggs Creamed Spinach with meatballs Smoothie					
Fasting 7pm – 4am	Green tea with Lemon					
Fasting _____						
Feeding _____						
Fasting _____						

Date

Last Bite Eaten @

Water

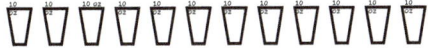

120 oz.

TO DO LIST

_____

_____

Workout Focus

Chest   Arms   Back   Legs   Abs   Cardio   Rest

                        ✓   ✓

I am so grateful for movement

Workouts in Reference

Workout Log

Exercise	Minutes	Reps	Weight	Sets
Elliptical	25	1		3
Body weight squat		20-30		3
Dumbbell lunges		15		3
Standing dumbbell calf raise		30-50		3
Crunches		30-50		3
Tuck Crunch		30-50		3

Notes

_____

_____

_____

_____

_____

_____

_____

_____

EXAMPLE

Day # 3 _____

Date

Nutrition

Window	Item	Calories	Fat (g)	Carb (g)	Fiber (g)	Protein (g)
Fasting 4am – 11 am	Green tea with Lemon					
Feeding 11am – 7pm	Eggs Creamed Spinach with meatballs Smoothie					
Fasting 7pm – 4am	Green tea with Lemon					
Fasting _____						
Feeding _____						
Fasting _____						

EXAMPLE

Last Bite Eaten @

Water

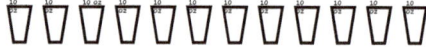

120 oz.

TO DO LIST

_____
_____

Workout Focus

Chest	Arms	Back	Glutes	Shoulder	Abs	Rest
✔	✔	✔		✔		

I am so grateful for movement

Workouts in Reference

Workout Log

Note

Exercise	Minutes	Reps	Weight	Sets
Elliptical	25	1		3
Barbell bench press		4-6		3
One Arm dumbbell row		4-6		3
Standing military press		4-6		3
Barbell Curl		4-6		3
Tricep Kickback		4-6		3

_____
_____
_____
_____
_____
_____
_____
_____
_____

Day # 4 _____

EXAMPLE

Date

Nutrition

Window	Item	Calories	Fat (g)	Carb (g)	Fiber (g)	Protein (g)
Fasting 4am – 11 am	Green tea with Lemon					
Feeding 11am – 7pm	Eggs Creamed Spinach with meatballs Smoothie					
Fasting 7pm – 4am	Green tea with Lemon					
Fasting _____						
Feeding _____						
Fasting _____						

Last Bite Eaten @

Water

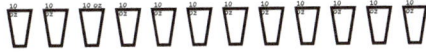

120 oz.

TO DO LIST

_____

_____

Workout Focus

Chest   Arms   Back   Glutes   Shoulder   Abs   Rest

I am so grateful for movement

Workouts in Reference

Workout Log

Notes

Exercise	Minutes	Reps	Weight	Sets
Yoga or Stretch	60			

_____

_____

_____

_____

_____

_____

_____

_____

Day # 5 _____

Nutrition

Window	Item	Calories	Fat (g)	Carb (g)	Fiber (g)	Protein (g)
Fasting 4am – 11 am	Green tea with Lemon					
Feeding 11am – 7pm	Eggs Creamed Spinach with meatballs Smoothie					
Fasting 7pm – 4am	Green tea with Lemon					
Fasting _____						
Feeding						
Fasting _____						

Date

EXAMPLE

Last Bite Eaten @

Water

120 oz.

TO DO LIST

_____
_____

Workout Focus

Chest   Arms   Back   Glutes ✓   Shoulder ✓   Abs   Rest

Workouts in Reference

I am so grateful for movement

Workout Log

Note

Exercise	Minutes	Reps	Weight	Sets
Elliptical	25	1		3
Body weight squat		20-30		3
Dumbbell lunges		15		3
Standing dumbbell calf raise		30-50		3
Crunches		30-50		3
Tuck Crunch		30-50		3

_____
_____
_____
_____
_____
_____
_____
_____

Day # 6 _____

Nutrition

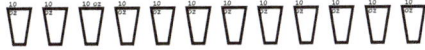

Date

Window	Item	Calories	Fat (g)	Carb (g)	Fiber (g)	Protein (g)
Fasting 4am – 11 am	Green tea with Lemon					
Feeding 11am – 7pm	Eggs Creamed Spinach with meatballs Smoothie					
Fasting 7pm – 4am	Green tea with Lemon					
Fasting _____						
Feeding _____						
Fasting _____						

EXAMPLE

Last Bite Eaten @

Water

🥤🥤🥤🥤🥤🥤🥤🥤🥤🥤🥤🥤

120 oz.

TO DO LIST

_____

_____

Workout Focus

Chest   Arms   Back   Glutes   Shoulder   Abs   Rest

I am so grateful for movement

Workouts in Reference

Workout Log

Notes

Exercise	Minutes	Reps	Weight	Sets
Active Recovery Rest				

_____
_____
_____
_____
_____
_____
_____
_____

Day # 7 _____

Nutrition

Window	Item	Calories	Fat (g)	Carb (g)	Fiber (g)	Protein (g)
Fasting 4am – 11 am	Green tea with Lemon					
Feeding 11am – 7pm	Eggs Creamed Spinach with meatballs Smoothie					
Fasting 7pm – 4am	Green tea with Lemon					
Fasting _____						
Feeding						
Fasting _____						

EXAMPLE

Last Bite Eaten @

Water

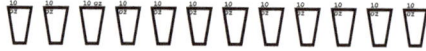

120 oz.

TO DO LIST

_____

_____

Workout Focus

Chest   Arms   Back   Glutes   Shoulder   Abs   Rest

Workouts in Reference

I am so grateful for movement

Workout Log

Exercise	Minutes	Reps	Weight	Sets
STRONG by Zumba	60			

Note

_____
_____
_____
_____
_____
_____
_____
_____
_____

Day # 8 _____

Nutrition

Window	Item	Calories	Fat (g)	Carb (g)	Fiber (g)	Protein (g)
Fasting 4am – 11 am	Green tea with Lemon					
Feeding 11am – 7pm	Eggs Creamed Spinach with meatballs Smoothie					
Fasting 7pm – 4am	Green tea with Lemon					
Fasting _____						
Feeding _____						
Fasting _____						

EXAMPLE

Last Bite Eaten @

Water
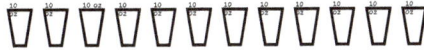

120 oz.

TO DO LIST
_____
_____

Workout Focus

Chest	Arms	Back	Glutes	Shoulder	Abs	Rest
✔	✔	✔		✔		

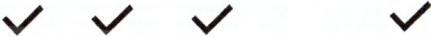

Workouts in Reference

I am so grateful for movement

Workout Log

Exercise	Minutes	Reps	Weight	Sets
Elliptical	25	1		3
Barbell bench press		4-6		3
One Arm dumbbell row		4-6		3
Standing military press		4-6		3
Barbell Curl		4-6		3
Tricep Kickback		4-6		3

Notes
_____
_____
_____
_____
_____
_____
_____
_____
_____

Day # 9 _____

Nutrition

Window	Item	Calories	Fat (g)	Carb (g)	Fiber (g)	Protein (g)
Fasting 4am – 11 am	Green tea with Lemon					
Feeding 11am – 7pm	Eggs Creamed Spinach with meatballs Smoothie					
Fasting 7pm – 4am	Green tea with Lemon					
Fasting _____						
Feeding _____						
Fasting _____						

EXAMPLE

Last Bite Eaten @

Water

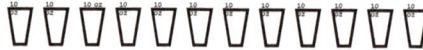

10 10 10 10 10 10 10 10 10 10 10 10

120 oz.

TO DO LIST

_____

_____

Workout Focus

Chest   Arms   Back   Legs   Abs   Cardio   Rest

✔   ✔

I am so grateful for movement

Workouts in Reference

Workout Log

Note

Exercise	Minutes	Reps	Weight	Sets
Elliptical	25	1		3
Body weight squat		20-30		3
Dumbbell lunges		15		3
Standing dumbbell calf raise		30-50		3
Crunches		30-50		3
Tuck Crunch		30-50		3

_____
_____
_____
_____
_____
_____
_____
_____

Day # 10 _____

Nutrition

Window	Item	Calories	Fat (g)	Carb (g)	Fiber (g)	Protein (g)
Fasting 4am – 11 am	Green tea with Lemon					
Feeding 11am – 7pm	Eggs Creamed Spinach with meatballs Smoothie					
Fasting 7pm – 4am	Green tea with Lemon					
Fasting _____						
Feeding _____						
Fasting _____						

EXAMPLE

Last Bite Eaten @

Water

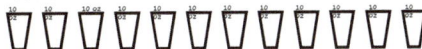

120 oz.

TO DO LIST

_____

_____

Workout Focus

Chest ✓   Arms ✓   Back ✓   Glutes   Shoulder ✓   Abs   Rest

Workouts in Reference

I am so grateful for movement

Workout Log

Notes

Exercise	Minutes	Reps	Weight	Sets
Elliptical	25	1		3
Barbell bench press		4-6		3
One Arm dumbbell row		4-6		3
Standing military press		4-6		3
Barbell Curl		4-6		3
Tricep Kickback		4-6		3

_____

_____

_____

_____

_____

_____

Day # 11 _____

Nutrition

Window	Item	Calories	Fat (g)	Carb (g)	Fiber (g)	Protein (g)
Fasting 4am – 11 am	Green tea with Lemon					
Feeding 11am – 7pm	Eggs Creamed Spinach with meatballs Smoothie					
Fasting 7pm – 4am	Green tea with Lemon					
Fasting _____						
Feeding _____						
Fasting _____						

EXAMPLE

Last Bite Eaten @

Water

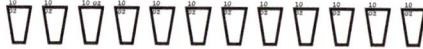

120 oz.

TO DO LIST

_____

_____

Workout Focus

Chest   Arms   Back   Glutes   Shoulder   Abs   Rest

Workouts in Reference

I am so grateful for movement

Workout Log

Exercise	Minutes	Reps	Weight	Sets
Yoga or Stretch	60			

Note

_____

_____

_____

_____

_____

_____

_____

_____

Day # 12 _____

Nutrition

Window	Item	Calories	Fat (g)	Carb (g)	Fiber (g)	Protein (g)
Fasting 4am – 11 am	Green tea with Lemon					
Feeding 11am – 7pm	Eggs Creamed Spinach with meatballs Smoothie					
Fasting 7pm – 4am	Green tea with Lemon					
Fasting _____						
Feeding _____						
Fasting _____						

EXAMPLE

Last Bite Eaten @

Water

120 oz.

TO DO LIST

_____
_____

Workout Focus

Chest   Arms   Back   Legs   Abs   Cardio   Rest
                          ✓   ✓

Workouts in Reference

I am so grateful for movement

Workout Log

Exercise	Minutes	Reps	Weight	Sets
Elliptical	25	1		3
Body weight squat		20-30		3
Dumbbell lunges		15		3
Standing dumbbell calf raise		30-50		3
Crunches		30-50		3
Tuck Crunch		30-50		3

Notes

_____
_____
_____
_____
_____
_____
_____
_____

Day # 13 _____

Nutrition

Window	Item	Calories	Fat (g)	Carb (g)	Fiber (g)	Protein (g)
Fasting 4am – 11 am	Green tea with Lemon					
Feeding 11am – 7pm	Eggs Creamed Spinach with meatballs Smoothie					
Fasting 7pm – 4am	Green tea with Lemon					
Fasting _____						
Feeding _____						
Fasting _____						

Date

EXAMPLE

Last Bite Eaten @

Water

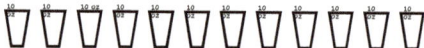

10 10 10 10 10 10 10 10 10 10 10 10

120 oz.

TO DO LIST

_____

_____

Workout Focus

Chest   Arms   Back   Glutes   Shoulder   Abs   Rest

I am so grateful for movement

Workouts in Reference

Workout Log

Exercise	Minutes	Reps	Weight	Sets
Active Recovery Rest				

Note

_____
_____
_____
_____
_____
_____
_____
_____
_____

Day # 14 _____

Date

Nutrition

Window	Item	Calories	Fat (g)	Carb (g)	Fiber (g)	Protein (g)
Fasting 4am – 11 am	Green tea with Lemon					
Feeding 11am – 7pm	Eggs Creamed Spinach with meatballs Smoothie					
Fasting 7pm – 4am	Green tea with Lemon					
Fasting _____						
Feeding _____						
Fasting _____						

EXAMPLE

Last Bite Eaten @   Water

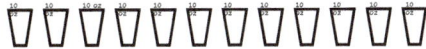

120 oz.

TO DO LIST

_____
_____

Workout Focus

Chest   Arms   Back   Glutes   Shoulder   Abs   Rest

I am so grateful for movement

Workouts in Reference

Workout Log

Notes

Exercise	Minutes	Reps	Weight	Sets
STRONG by Zumba	60			

_____
_____
_____
_____
_____
_____
_____
_____
_____

Day # 15 _____

Nutrition

Window	Item	Calories	Fat (g)	Carb (g)	Fiber (g)	Protein (g)
Fasting 4am – 11 am	Green tea with Lemon					
Feeding 11am – 7pm	Eggs Creamed Spinach with meatballs Smoothie					
Fasting 7pm – 4am	Green tea with Lemon					
Fasting _____						
Feeding _____						
Fasting _____						

EXAMPLE

Last Bite Eaten @

Water

🥤 10 🥤 10 🥤 oz 🥤 10 🥤 10 🥤 10 🥤 10 🥤 10 🥤 10 🥤 10 🥤 10 🥤 10

120 oz.

TO DO LIST

_____
_____

Workout Focus

Chest	Arms	Back	Glutes	Shoulder	Abs	Rest
✓	✓	✓		✓		

Workouts in Reference

I am so grateful for movement

Workout Log

Exercise	Minutes	Reps	Weight	Sets
. Elliptical	25	1		3
Barbell bench press		4-6		3
One Arm dumbbell row		4-6		3
Standing military press		4-6		3
Barbell Curl		4-6		3
Tricep Kickback		4-6		3

Note

_____
_____
_____
_____
_____
_____
_____
_____
_____

Day # 16 _____

Date _____

Window	Item	Calories	Fat (g)	Carb (g)	Fiber (g)	Protein (g)
Fasting 4am – 11 am	Green tea with Lemon					
Feeding 11am – 7pm	Eggs Creamed Spinach with meatballs Smoothie					
Fasting 7pm – 4am	Green tea with Lemon					
Fasting _____						
Feeding _____						
Fasting _____						

EXAMPLE

Last Bite Eaten @

Water

120 oz.

TO DO LIST

_____

_____

Workout Focus

Chest   Arms   Back   Legs   Abs   Cardio   Rest

                            ✓   ✓

Workouts in Reference

I am so grateful for movement

Workout Log

Notes

Exercise	Minutes	Reps	Weight	Sets
Elliptical	25	1		3
Body weight squat		20-30		3
Dumbbell lunges		15		3
Standing dumbbell calf raise		30-50		3
Crunches		30-50		3
Tuck Crunch		30-50		3

_____

_____

_____

_____

_____

_____

_____

_____

Day # 17 _____

Date

Nutrition

Window	Item	Calories	Fat (g)	Carb (g)	Fiber (g)	Protein (g)
Fasting 4am – 11 am	Green tea with Lemon					
Feeding 11am – 7pm	Eggs Creamed Spinach with meatballs Smoothie					
Fasting 7pm – 4am	Green tea with Lemon					
Fasting _____						
Feeding _____						
Fasting _____						

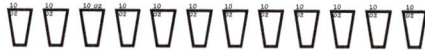

Last Bite Eaten @

Water

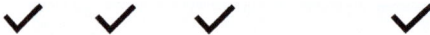

120 oz.

TO DO LIST

_____

_____

Workout Focus

Chest	Arms	Back	Glutes	Shoulder	Abs	Rest
✓	✓	✓		✓		

Workouts in Reference

I am so grateful for movement

Workout Log

Exercise	Minutes	Reps	Weight	Sets
Elliptical	25	1		3
Barbell bench press		4-6		3
One Arm dumbbell row		4-6		3
Standing military press		4-6		3
Barbell Curl		4-6		3
Tricep Kickback		4-6		3

Note

_____

_____

_____

_____

_____

_____

_____

_____

Day # 18 _____

Nutrition

Window	Item	Calories	Fat (g)	Carb (g)	Fiber (g)	Protein (g)
Fasting 4am – 11 am	Green tea with Lemon					
Feeding 11am – 7pm	Eggs Creamed Spinach with meatballs Smoothie					
Fasting 7pm – 4am	Green tea with Lemon					
Fasting _____						
Feeding _____						
Fasting _____						

Date

EXAMPLE

Last Bite Eaten @

Water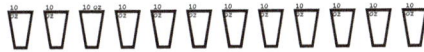

120 oz.

TO DO LIST

_____
_____

Workout Focus

Chest   Arms   Back   Glutes   Shoulder   Abs   Rest

I am so grateful for movement

Workouts in Reference

Workout Log

Notes

Exercise	Minutes	Reps	Weight	Sets
Yoga or Stretch	60			

_____
_____
_____
_____
_____
_____
_____
_____

Day # 19 _____

Nutrition

Window	Item	Calories	Fat (g)	Carb (g)	Fiber (g)	Protein (g)
Fasting 4am – 11 am	Green tea with Lemon					
Feeding 11am – 7pm	Eggs Creamed Spinach with meatballs Smoothie					
Fasting 7pm – 4am	Green tea with Lemon					
Fasting _____						
Feeding _____						
Fasting _____						

EXAMPLE

Last Bite Eaten @

Water

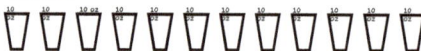

120 oz.

TO DO LIST

_____

_____

Workout Focus

Chest   Arms   Back   Glutes   Shoulder   Abs   Rest

Workouts in Reference

I am so grateful for movement

Workout Log

Note

Exercise	Minutes	Reps	Weight	Sets
Elliptical	25	1		3
Body weight squat		20-30		3
Dumbbell lunges		15		3
Standing dumbbell calf raise		30-50		3
Crunches		30-50		3
Tuck Crunch		30-50		3

_____

_____

_____

_____

_____

_____

_____

_____

Day # 20 _____

Nutrition

Window	Item	Calories	Fat (g)	Carb (g)	Fiber (g)	Protein (g)
Fasting 4am – 11 am	Green tea with Lemon					
Feeding 11am – 7pm	Eggs Creamed Spinach with meatballs Smoothie					
Fasting 7pm – 4am	Green tea with Lemon					
Fasting _____						
Feeding _____						
Fasting _____						

EXAMPLE

Date

Last Bite Eaten @

Water 10 oz (×12 glasses)

120 oz.

TO DO LIST

_____
_____

Workout Focus

Chest   Arms   Back   Glutes   Shoulder   Abs   Rest

Workouts in Reference

I am so grateful for movement

Workout Log

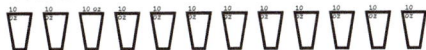

<u>Notes</u>

Exercise	Minutes	Reps	Weight	Sets
Active Recovery Rest				

_____
_____
_____
_____
_____
_____
_____
_____
_____
_____

Day # 21 _____

Nutrition

Window	Item	Calories	Fat (g)	Carb (g)	Fiber (g)	Protein (g)
Fasting 4am – 11 am	Green tea with Lemon					
Feeding 11am – 7pm	Eggs Creamed Spinach with meatballs Smoothie					
Fasting 7pm – 4am	Green tea with Lemon					
Fasting _____						
Feeding _____						
Fasting _____						

EXAMPLE

Last Bite Eaten @

Water
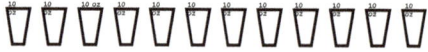

120 oz.

TO DO LIST

_____
_____

Workout Focus

Chest   Arms   Back   Glutes   Shoulder   Abs   Rest

Workouts in Reference

I am so grateful for movement

Workout Log

Exercise	Minutes	Reps	Weight	Sets
STRONG by Zumba	60			

Note

_____
_____
_____
_____
_____
_____
_____
_____
_____

You made it!

How did you do?

How do you feel?

Did you learn something about yourself?

Get that tape measure back out and update your progress on the next page. Make sure to check in with me and let's talk about your successes.

I am so proud of you and I look forward to supporting you in reaching your goals.

This was one cycle towards reaching your goals.

How did that commitment feel?

Want to continue moving forward?

Finish..........

Before:
I feel......
I improved in _____way .....
Proven by ....

This is me on _____(date).

I recommend that you attach a printed picture

Mid section

Arms

Lower body

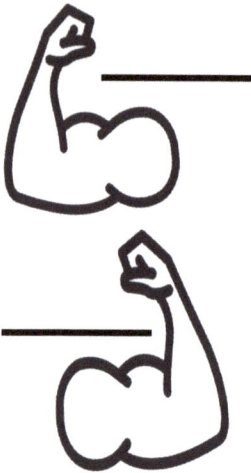

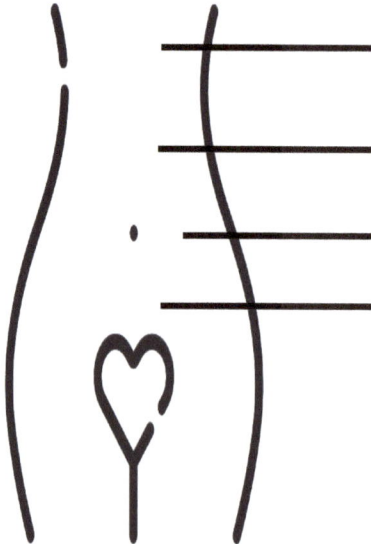

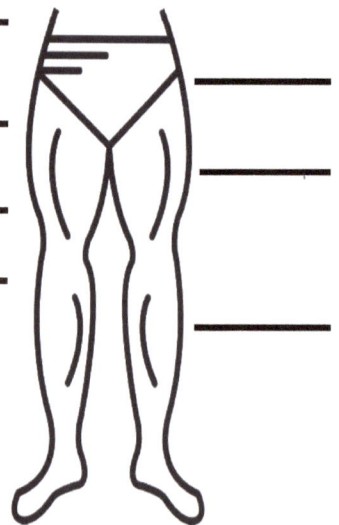

"Icon made by FreePik from www.flaticon.com"

"Icon made by FreePik from www.flaticon.com"

"Icon made by FreePik from www.flaticon.com"

In your head

Take some time to reflect on this experience. Take note of any

~ thoughts

~ gratitude

~ questions

~ concerns

Recipe Ideas for next cycle
~
Grocery list

Thank you!!!!

I hope your enjoyed this taste of the **My Portions** program and got the results you were expecting in this short time. This program can be staggered over longer time frames in cycles to meet long term nutritional goals. Personal training is supported by the **My Portions** program and is also tailored to meet your needs.

For more information, or to continue the program, please contact Our Others Keeper (OOK).

www.ingramcontent.com/pod-product-compliance
Lightning Source LLC
Chambersburg PA
CBHW041215270326
41930CB00001B/30